CONFLICT TO BLISS

The surprising path to deeper love

Charles C. Smith

INTRODUCTION

Welcome to Conflict to Bliss: The Surprising Path to Deeper Love

The Purpose and Scope of this Book

How to Use This Book to Transform Your Relationships

CHAPTER ONE: THE PARADOX OF CONFLICT

The Surprising Truth About Conflict in Relationships

Why We Fear Conflict (And Why We Shouldn't)

CHAPTER TWO: UNDERSTANDING THE ROOTS OF CONFLICTS

Uncovering the Hidden Patterns and Beliefs that Fuel Conflicts

How Unmet Needs and Unexpressed Emotions Create Tension

The Role of Power and Control in Relationship Conflict

CHAPTER THREE: THE ART OF CONFLICT TRANSFORMATION

Active Listening and Empathy: The Keys to Unlocking Understanding

How to Use Conflict to Build Intimacy and Trust

CHAPTER FOUR: NAVIGATING THE STORM

Strategies for Managing Intense Emotions and Escalating Conflicts

The Art of Apologizing and Forgiving: When and How to Do It

Finding the Lesson in the Conflict: Personal Growth and Self-Discovery

CHAPTER FIVE: BUILDING A CULTURE OF BLISS

Creating a Safe and Supportive Relationship Environment

The Power of Appreciation and Gratitude in Relationships

Sustaining Connection and Intimacy in the Long Term

CHAPTER SIX: PUTTING IT ALL TOGETHER

Conflict to Bliss: The Journey from Separation to Union

Maintaining Momentum and Embracing the Journey

EPILOGUE

The Surprising Path to Deeper Love: A Final Word

INTRODUCTION

Welcome to Conflict to Bliss: The Surprising Path to Deeper Love

Are you tired of feeling like conflicts are tearing your relationship apart? Do you long for a deeper connection with your partner, but don't know how to get past the arguments and disagreements? You're not alone. Conflict is a natural part of any relationship, but it doesn't have to be a source of pain and suffering. In fact, conflicts can be a catalyst for growth, understanding, and deeper love.

In this book, we'll explore the surprising ways that conflict can bring you closer together. We'll delve into the reasons why conflicts arise, and how they can be used as opportunities for growth and understanding. You'll learn how to communicate effectively, manage intense emotions, and find common ground, even in the most difficult situations.
Through personal anecdotes, real-life examples, and expert insights, we'll show you how to transform your conflicts into opportunities for deeper love and connection.

We'll take you on a journey of discovery, exploring the hidden dynamics of conflict and the secrets to resolving them in a way that strengthens your relationship.

Get ready to discover a new way of relating to your partner, one that embraces conflicts as a natural part of your journey together. Get ready to find bliss in the midst of conflict, and to emerge stronger, wiser, and more in love than ever before.

In the following pages, we'll explore the surprising truth about conflict in relationships, why we fear it, and how it can be a catalyst for growth and understanding. We'll delve into the roots of conflict, including hidden patterns, unmet needs, and power dynamics. We'll learn how to communicate effectively, manage intense emotions, and find common ground. We'll discover how to use conflict to build intimacy and trust, and how to create a safe and supportive relationship environment.

By the end of this journey, you'll have the tools and techniques you need to transform your conflicts into opportunities for deeper love and connection. You'll be able to navigate even the most challenging conflicts with.

The Purpose and Scope of this Book

This book is designed to be a transformative guide for couples who want to turn their conflicts into opportunities for growth, understanding, and deeper love.

The purpose of this book is to provide couples with the tools and techniques they need to transform their conflicts into a powerful tool for building a stronger, more loving relationship. We believe that conflicts are not something to be avoided or feared, but rather an opportunity for growth, understanding, and intimacy.

This book will cover a wide range of topics related to conflict resolution, communication, emotional intelligence, and building a strong and loving relationship. We will explore the surprising truth about conflict in relationships, why we fear it, and how it can be a catalyst for growth and understanding.

We will delve into the roots of conflict, including hidden patterns, unmet needs, and power dynamics. We will learn how to communicate effectively, manage intense emotions, and find common ground. We will discover how to use conflict to build intimacy and trust, and how to create a safe and supportive relationship environment.

Throughout this book, we will share personal anecdotes, real-life examples, and expert insights to help you navigate even the most challenging conflicts. We will provide practical strategies and techniques for transforming conflicts into opportunities for deeper love and connection.

By the end of this book, you will have the tools and techniques you need to:

- Understand the surprising truth about conflict in relationships
- Identify the roots of conflict and how to address them
- Communicate effectively and manage intense emotions
- Find common ground and build intimacy and trust
- Create a safe and supportive relationship environment

Get ready to transform your conflicts into a powerful tool for building a stronger, more loving relationship. Let's embark on this journey together!

How to Use This Book to Transform Your Relationships

Congratulations on taking the first step towards transforming your relationships! This book is designed to be a practical guide for couples who want to turn their conflicts into opportunities for growth, understanding, and deeper love.
To get the most out of this book, we recommend that you approach it with an open mind, a willingness to learn, and a commitment to taking action.

 Here are some tips on how to use this book to transform your relationships:

1. Read it together: This book is designed for couples, so we recommend that you read it together. Take turns reading chapters, discussing questions, and exploring exercises.

2. Be honest and vulnerable: Conflict transformation requires honesty and vulnerability. Be willing to confront your own flaws, fears, and insecurities.

3. Practice active listening: Listen carefully to your partner's perspective, and try to understand their needs, desires, and emotions.

4. Take responsibility: Conflicts are often a result of unmet needs, unresolved issues, or unexpressed emotions. Take responsibility for your part in the conflict.

5. Be patient and persistent: Conflict transformation takes time, effort, and practice. Don't expect to resolve everything overnight.

6. Use the exercises and questions: This book includes practical exercises and questions to help you apply the concepts to your relationship. Take the time to work through them.

7. Seek support: Consider seeking support from a therapist, counselor, or coach who can provide guidance and support.

By following these tips, you can use this book to transform your relationships and turn conflicts into opportunities for growth, understanding, and deeper love. Remember, conflict transformation is a journey, not a destination. It takes time, effort, and practice, but the rewards are well worth it.

Let's get started on this journey together!

CHAPTER ONE: THE PARADOX OF CONFLICT

The Surprising Truth About Conflict in Relationships

Conflict is a natural part of any relationship. It's an inevitable reality that can arise from differences in opinions, values, beliefs, and needs. Yet, despite its ubiquity, conflict is often viewed as a negative and destructive force that can tear relationships apart.

But what if we're looking at conflict the wrong way? What if, instead of being a source of pain and suffering, conflict is actually a catalyst for growth, understanding, and deeper love?

The surprising truth about conflict in relationships is that it's not something to be avoided or feared. Rather, it's an opportunity to be embraced and explored. By leaning into conflict, we can gain a deeper understanding of ourselves and our partners, and build stronger, more resilient relationships.

Conflict to Bliss

One of the most significant misconceptions about conflict is that it's a sign of a flawed or failing relationship. We often believe that if we're experiencing conflict, it means that we're not meant to be with our partner or that our relationship is somehow broken.

But the truth is that conflict is a natural part of any relationship. It's a sign that we're growing and evolving together and that we're willing to confront our differences and work through them.
Another misconception about conflict is that it's always negative and destructive. We often assume that conflict will lead to hurt feelings, damaged relationships, and even break-ups.

But the truth is that conflict can be a powerful tool for transformation. It can help us to confront our own flaws and weaknesses, to challenge our assumptions and biases, and to grow and evolve as individuals.

So, how can we begin to see conflict in this new light? How can we start to view conflict as an opportunity for growth and transformation, rather than a source of pain and suffering?

First, we need to recognize that conflict is a natural part of any relationship. It's not something that's wrong or abnormal, but rather a sign that we're growing and evolving together.

Second, we need to approach conflict with an open mind and a willingness to learn. This means being curious about our partner's perspective and seeking to understand their needs and desires.

Finally, we need to be willing to take risks and be vulnerable. This means being honest about our own flaws and weaknesses and being willing to confront our own biases and assumptions.

By embracing conflict as a natural part of our relationships, we can transform our conflicts into opportunities for growth, understanding, and deeper love. We can build stronger, more resilient relationships that are capable of withstanding even the most challenging conflicts.

So, the next time you find yourself in the midst of a conflict, remember that it's not something to be feared or avoided. Instead, it's an opportunity to be embraced and explored. By leaning into conflict, you can gain a deeper understanding of yourself and your partner, and build a stronger, more loving relationship.

Why We Fear Conflict (And Why We Shouldn't)

Conflict is a natural part of life, yet many of us fear it. We fear that conflict will lead to hurt feelings, damaged relationships, and even violence. But what if our fear of conflict is actually doing more harm than good we'll explore the reasons why we fear conflict and why we shouldn't. We'll examine the misconceptions and myths that surround conflict and discover the surprising benefits of embracing conflict.

Misconception 1: Conflict is always negative

One of the most significant misconceptions about conflict is that it's always negative. We often associate conflict with anger, aggression, and hurt feelings. However, conflict can also be a positive force for change, growth, and understanding.

Misconception 2: Conflict is a sign of weakness

We often believe that conflict is a sign of weakness, that we're not strong enough to handle our differences and work through them. But conflict takes courage, and it's a sign of strength to be willing to engage in difficult conversations and work toward a resolution.

Misconception 3: Conflict is a threat to relationships

We often fear that conflict will damage our relationships, but conflict can bring us closer together. When we work through conflicts, we build trust, understanding, and intimacy.

Misconception 4: Conflict is always about winning or losing

We often approach conflict as a competition, where one person wins and the other loses. But conflict is not a zero-sum game. It's possible to find a resolution that satisfies both parties.

The Benefits of Embracing Conflict

So, why should we embrace conflict? Here are just a few reasons:
1. Conflict promotes growth and understanding
2. Conflict builds trust and intimacy
3. Conflict fosters creativity and innovation
4. Conflict develops emotional intelligence and empathy
5. Conflict leads to personal and professional growth

Conflict is a natural part of life, and it's not something to be feared. By embracing conflict, we can build stronger relationships, promote growth and understanding, and develop emotional intelligence and empathy. Remember, conflict is not a sign of weakness, but a sign of strength. So, the next time you find yourself in a conflict, approach it with courage, curiosity, and an open mind. You might find that it leads to a breakthrough.

CHAPTER TWO: UNDERSTANDING THE ROOTS OF CONFLICTS

Uncovering the Hidden Patterns and Beliefs that Fuel Conflicts

Conflicts are an inevitable part of our personal and professional lives. They can arise from differences in opinions, values, beliefs, and needs. However, often, conflicts are not just about the surface-level issues, but about the underlying patterns and beliefs that fuel them. We will explore the hidden patterns and beliefs that fuel conflicts and how to uncover them.

Hidden Pattern 1: The Need to Be Right

One of the most common hidden patterns that fuel conflicts is the need to be right. This pattern is driven by a deep-seated belief that our perspective is the only correct one and that others are wrong. When we are driven by this need, we become entrenched in our position and are unwilling to listen to others or consider alternative perspectives.

Hidden Pattern 2: The Fear of Vulnerability

Another hidden pattern that fuels conflicts is the fear of vulnerability. This pattern is driven by a belief that showing vulnerability is a sign of weakness and that others will take advantage of us if we are vulnerable. When we are driven by this fear, we become defensive and closed off, making it difficult to resolve conflicts.

Hidden Pattern 3: The Belief in Scarcity

The belief in scarcity is another hidden pattern that fuels conflicts. This pattern is driven by a belief that there is not enough to go around and that others are competing with us for resources. When we are driven by this belief, we become competitive and aggressive, leading to conflicts.

Hidden Pattern 4: The Need for Control

The need for control is another hidden pattern that fuels conflicts. This pattern is driven by a belief that we need to control others and our environment in order to feel safe and secure. When we are driven by this need, we become domineering and manipulative, leading to conflicts.

Uncovering Hidden Patterns and Beliefs

So, how can we uncover these hidden patterns and beliefs that fuel conflicts? Here are a few strategies:

1. Self-reflection: Take time to reflect on your thoughts, feelings, and behaviors in conflicts. What are your triggers? What are your go-to responses?

2. Active listening: Listen carefully to others in conflicts. What are their underlying concerns and needs?

3. Inquiry: Ask questions to uncover the underlying patterns and beliefs that are driving the conflict.

4. Mindfulness: Practice mindfulness to become more aware of your thoughts, feelings, and behaviors in conflicts.

Breaking Free from Hidden Patterns and Beliefs

Once we have uncovered the hidden patterns and beliefs that fuel conflicts, we can begin to break free from them. Here are a few strategies:

1. Challenge negative self-talk: Challenge negative self-talk and replace it with more positive and realistic thoughts.

2. Practice empathy: Practice empathy and understanding towards others.

3. Develop a growth mindset: Develop a growth mindset and be open to learning and growing.

4. Seek support: Seek support from others, such as therapists or coaches, to help us break free from hidden patterns and beliefs.

Conflicts are an inevitable part of our lives, but they don't have to be debilitating. By uncovering the hidden patterns and beliefs that fuel conflicts, we can begin to break free from them and develop more constructive ways of relating to ourselves and others. Remember, conflicts are opportunities for growth and learning, and by uncovering the hidden patterns and beliefs that fuel them, we can become more aware, more empathetic, and more effective in our personal and professional lives.

How Unmet Needs and Unexpressed Emotions Create Tension

Have you ever felt like you're walking on eggshells around your partner, never knowing when they'll blow up or shut down? Or maybe you're the one who's always simmering with resentment, feeling like your needs are never met. Tension in relationships is a ubiquitous phenomenon, and it's often caused by two underlying issues: unmet needs and unexpressed emotions.

Let's delve into the world of unmet needs and unexpressed emotions, exploring how they create tension in relationships and what you can do to break the cycle.

Unmet Needs: The Silent Killer of Relationships

Unmet needs are the foundation of tension in relationships. When our needs are not met, we feel frustrated, resentful, and angry. We may even feel like we're not being seen or heard by our partners. Unmet needs can arise from various aspects of a relationship, including emotional, physical, and intellectual needs.

Emotional needs include feeling loved, appreciated, and validated. Physical needs encompass intimacy, touch, and affection. Intellectual needs involve being understood, respected, and stimulated. When these needs are not met, tension arises, and conflict ensues.

Unexpressed Emotions: The Pressure Cooker of Tension

Unexpressed emotions are another significant contributor to tension in relationships. When we don't express our emotions, they build up inside us, creating pressure and stress. This pressure cooker of emotions can lead to explosive conflicts or passive-aggressive behavior.

Unexpressed emotions can stem from various sources, including fear, shame, guilt, or vulnerability. We may feel uncomfortable expressing our emotions due to past experiences, cultural conditioning, or fear of rejection. However, bottling up emotions only exacerbates tension and can lead to emotional numbness.

The Consequences of Unmet Needs and Unexpressed Emotions

The consequences of unmet needs and unexpressed emotions can be devastating. Tension builds up, causing conflicts to escalate and relationships to deteriorate. We may feel disconnected, unheard, and unvalidated. In extreme cases, unmet needs and unexpressed emotions can lead to emotional or physical abuse.

Breaking the Cycle of Tension

So, how can you break the cycle of tension caused by unmet needs and unexpressed emotions? The answer lies in communication, empathy, and self-awareness.

1. Identify Your Needs and Emotions

Start by recognizing your unmet needs and unexpressed emotions. Take time to reflect on what you're feeling and what you need from your partner. Be honest with yourself, and don't be afraid to explore your emotions.

2. Communicate Your Needs and Emotions

Once you've identified your needs and emotions, communicate them to your partner. Use "I" statements to express your feelings and avoid blaming or accusing your partner. Be specific about what you need and how you feel.

3. Listen to Your Partner's Needs and Emotions

Listening is a crucial aspect of breaking the cycle of tension. When your partner expresses their needs and emotions, listen actively and empathetically. Avoid interrupting or dismissing their feelings. Show that you understand and care about their needs.

4. Validate Each Other's Needs and Emotions
Validation is essential in relationships. When you validate your partner's needs and emotions, you show that you respect and understand them. This helps to create a safe and supportive environment where both partners feel heard and seen.

5. Find Common Ground
Finally, find common ground by compromising and finding solutions that meet both partners' needs. Be willing to negotiate and find creative solutions that satisfy both parties.

Unmet needs and unexpressed emotions are the silent killers of relationships. They create tension, conflict, and disconnection. However, by recognizing and addressing these issues, you can break the cycle of tension and create a more harmonious and fulfilling relationship. Remember to communicate your needs and emotions, listen to your partner, validate each other's feelings, and find common ground. By doing so, you'll be well on your way to building a stronger, more loving relationship.

The Role of Power and Control in Relationship Conflict

Relationship conflict is a natural part of any partnership. However, when power and control are at play, conflict can become a recurring and debilitating pattern. In this article, we'll explore the role of power and control in relationship conflict and how it can affect our relationships.

What is Power and Control in Relationships?

Power and control in relationships refer to the ability of one partner to influence and dominate the other partner's thoughts, feelings, and actions. This can manifest in various ways, such as financial control, emotional manipulation, and physical coercion.

Types of Power and Control

There are several types of power and control that can manifest in relationships, including:

1. Covert power: This type of power is exercised through subtle and indirect means, such as guilt-tripping, gaslighting, and emotional blackmail.

2. Overt power: This type of power is exercised through direct and obvious means, such as physical violence, verbal abuse, and financial control.

3. Cultural power: This type of power is exercised through cultural norms and expectations, such as gender roles and social status.

How Power and Control Affect Relationship Conflict

Power and control can significantly affect relationship conflict in several ways:

1. Creates resentment: When one partner feels controlled or dominated, they may feel resentful and angry, leading to conflict.

2. Fosters fear: Power and control can create a culture of fear, where one partner is afraid to express their needs and feelings.

3. Limits communication: Power and control can limit open and honest communication, leading to misunderstandings and conflict.

4. Increases tension: Power and control can create tension and stress in a relationship, leading to conflict.

Breaking the Cycle of Power and Control

So, how can we break the cycle of power and control in our relationships? Here are a few strategies:

1. Identify and challenge harmful power dynamics: Take time to reflect on your relationship and identify any harmful power dynamics.

2. Practice mutual respect: Treat your partner with respect and dignity, and expect the same in return.

3. Communicate openly and honestly: Practice open and honest communication to avoid misunderstandings and conflict.

4. Seek support: Consider couples therapy or counseling to work through power and control issues.

5. Empower each other: Share power and control, and support each other's autonomy.

Power and control can significantly affect relationship conflict. By understanding the types of power and control, how they affect relationship conflict, and breaking the cycle of power and control, we can build.

CHAPTER THREE: THE ART OF CONFLICT TRANSFORMATION

Active Listening and Empathy: The Keys to Unlocking Understanding

In today's fast-paced world, communication is more important than ever. With the rise of technology, we are constantly connected to others, but are we truly communicating? Or are we just existing in a state of constant distraction?

Effective communication is the foundation of any successful relationship, be it personal or professional. At the heart of effective communication are two essential skills: active listening and empathy.

we will explore the importance of active listening and empathy in unlocking understanding and building strong relationships. We will also discuss practical tips and strategies for improving your active listening and empathy skills.

The Importance of Active Listening

Active listening is the process of fully concentrating on what someone is saying, understanding their perspective, and responding in a thoughtful and engaged manner. It's about being present in the moment and giving the speaker your undivided attention.

Active listening is important because it helps to:

- Build trust and rapport with others
- Understand different perspectives and points of view
- Resolve conflicts and misunderstandings
- Improve communication and reduce errors
- Show respect and empathy towards others

The Importance of Empathy

Empathy is the ability to understand and share the feelings of others. It's about putting yourself in someone else's shoes and seeing things from their perspective.

Empathy is important because it helps to:

- Build strong relationships and connections with others
- Understand and respond to the emotional needs of others
- Create a safe and supportive environment for others to open up and share their feelings
- Improve communication and reduce conflicts
- Show compassion and understanding towards others

Practical Tips and Strategies for Improving Active Listening and Empathy Skills

Here are some practical tips and strategies for improving your active listening and empathy skills:

- Give the speaker your undivided attention and avoid distractions
- Use verbal and nonverbal cues to show you're engaged and interested
- Paraphrase and summarize what the speaker has said to ensure understanding
- Ask open-ended questions to encourage the speaker to share more
- Practice mindfulness and self-reflection to improve your emotional intelligence
- Put yourself in others' shoes and try to see things from their perspective
- Show compassion and understanding towards others and validate their feelings

Active listening and empathy are essential skills for effective communication and building strong relationships. By practicing these skills, you can improve your understanding of others, build trust and rapport, and create a safe and supportive environment for others to open up and share their feelings. Remember, effective communication is the foundation of any successful relationship, and active listening and empathy are the keys to unlocking understanding.

How to Use Conflict to Build Intimacy and Trust

Conflict is a natural part of any relationship. Two people with different backgrounds, experiences, and perspectives will inevitably disagree on certain things. However, conflict doesn't have to be a negative force that drives people apart. Instead, it can be a powerful tool for building intimacy and trust.

We will be exploring how conflict can be used to strengthen relationships and create a deeper sense of connection with others. We'll also discuss practical strategies for navigating conflicts in a way that fosters intimacy and trust.

The Surprising Benefits of Conflict

While conflict is often seen as a negative force, it has several surprising benefits. For one, conflict can help to:

- Clarify expectations and needs
- Build trust and intimacy
- Foster creativity and problem-solving
- Promote personal growth and self-awareness
- Strengthen relationships and bonds

How Conflict Can Build Intimacy

Conflict can help to build intimacy in several ways:

- By forcing us to communicate more openly and honestly
- By requiring us to listen more actively and empathetically

- By encouraging us to be more vulnerable and authentic

- By helping us to develop a deeper understanding of each other's needs and desires

- By fostering a sense of mutual respect and trust
How Conflict Can Build Trust

Conflict can also help to build trust in several ways:

- By providing opportunities for us to follow through on our commitments

- By requiring us to be more reliable

- By encouraging us to be more transparent and accountable

- By helping us to develop a sense of mutual support and loyalty

- By fostering a sense of fairness and justice
Practical Strategies for Navigating Conflict

Here are some practical strategies for navigating conflict in a way that fosters intimacy and trust:

- Approach conflicts with an open and non-defensive mindset

- Listen actively and empathetically to the other person's perspective

- Communicate openly and honestly about your own needs and feelings

- Seek common ground and compromise

- Be willing to apologize and forgive

- Show appreciation and gratitude for the other person's perspective

- Take breaks and practice self-care when needed

Conflict is a natural part of any relationship, but it doesn't have to be a negative force that drives people apart. Instead, it can be a powerful tool for building intimacy and trust. By approaching conflicts with an open and non-defensive mindset, listening actively and empathetically, communicating openly and honestly, seeking common ground and compromise, being willing to apologize and forgive, showing appreciation and gratitude, and taking breaks and practicing self-care when needed, we can use conflict to strengthen our relationships and create a deeper sense of connection with others.

Remember, conflict is not something to be feared or avoided, but rather something to be embraced and leveraged as a powerful tool for building intimacy and trust.

CHAPTER FOUR: NAVIGATING THE STORM

Strategies for Managing Intense Emotions and Escalating Conflicts

Intense emotions and escalating conflicts are a natural part of life, but they can be overwhelming and destructive if not managed properly. In this chapter, we will explore strategies for managing intense emotions and escalating conflicts healthily and constructively.

Understanding Intense Emotions

Intense emotions are normal and necessary for our well-being. They help us to respond to threats, pursue our goals, and build strong relationships. However, when intense emotions are not managed properly, they can lead to conflict, harm relationships, and even damage our physical and mental health.

Strategies for Managing Intense Emotions

Here are some strategies for managing intense emotions:

1. Identify and label your emotions: Recognize how you are feeling and give your emotions a name. This helps to process and release your emotions.
2. Take a time-out: Sometimes, we need to step away from a situation to calm down and reflect on our emotions.

3. Practice self-care: Take care of your physical, emotional, and mental health by getting enough sleep, exercising regularly, and engaging in activities that bring you joy and relaxation.

4. Use positive self-talk: Encourage yourself with positive affirmations and challenge negative self-talk.

5. Seek social support: Talk to a trusted friend, family member, or mental health professional about your emotions and receive support and guidance.

Understanding Escalating Conflicts

Escalating conflicts are a natural part of life, but they can be destructive if not managed properly. Conflicts can arise from differences in opinions, values, and needs, and can be escalated by poor communication, defensiveness, and a lack of empathy.

Strategies for Managing Escalating Conflicts

Here are some strategies for managing escalating conflicts:

1. Stay calm and composed: Manage your emotions and respond thoughtfully to the situation.
2. Practice active listening: Listen carefully to the other person's perspective and respond with empathy and understanding.

3. Use "I" statements: Express your feelings and needs using "I" statements, which help to avoid blame and defensiveness.

4. Seek common ground: Look for areas of agreement and try to find a mutually beneficial solution.

5. Take a break: Sometimes, it's necessary to take a break from a conflict to calm down and reflect on the situation.

Managing intense emotions and escalating conflicts is a vital skill for maintaining healthy relationships, achieving personal growth, and promoting overall well-being. By understanding and labeling our emotions, practicing self-care, seeking social support, staying calm and composed, practicing active listening, using "I" statements, seeking common ground, and taking breaks when needed, we can manage intense emotions and escalating conflicts healthily and constructively.

Remember, conflicts are opportunities for growth, learning, and deeper understanding, and by managing them effectively, we can build stronger, more resilient relationships and achieve greater personal fulfillment.

The Art of Apologizing and Forgiving: When and How to Do It

Apologizing and forgiving are two of the most powerful tools we have for building and maintaining strong, healthy relationships. Yet, many of us struggle with when and how to use them effectively.

we will explore the art of apologizing and forgiving, including when and how to do it, and why it's so important for our personal and professional relationships.

The Power of Apologizing

Apologizing is a powerful way to show respect, empathy, and understanding towards others. When we apologize, we take responsibility for our actions and show that we value the other person's feelings and well-being.

Here are some reasons why apologizing is so important:

- It shows that we value the other person's feelings and well-being
- It takes the focus off of our ego and defenses
- It helps to diffuse tension and conflict
- It builds trust and credibility
- It shows that we are willing to learn and grow from our mistakes

The Art of Apologizing

So, how do we apologize effectively? Here are some tips:

- Use the "3 Rs" of apologizing: regret, responsibility, and remedy
- Be sincere and genuine in your apology
- Use "I" statements to take ownership of your actions
- Be specific about what you are apologizing for
- Listen to the other person's perspective and validate their feelings
- Offer a solution or make amends if possible

The Power of Forgiving

Forgiving is a powerful way to let go of negative emotions and move forward in a positive direction. When we forgive, we release the hold that the other person has on us, and we take back control of our own emotions and well-being.

Here are some reasons why forgiving is so important:

- It releases negative emotions and energy
- It takes the focus off of the other person's actions and puts it back on ourselves
- It helps to heal and move forward
- It builds self-esteem and confidence
- It shows that we are willing to let go of the past and move forward

The Art of Forgiving

So, how do we forgive effectively? Here are some tips:

- Let go of the need to be right or to win
- Practice empathy and understanding towards the other person
- Use "I" statements to take ownership of your feelings and actions
- Be specific about what you are forgiving
- Take care of yourself and prioritize your well-being
- Seek support from others if needed

Apologizing and forgiving are two of the most powerful tools we have for building and maintaining strong, healthy relationships. By understanding when and how to use them effectively, we can build trust, credibility, and stronger relationships. Remember, apologizing and forgiving are not always easy, but it's worth it in the end.

Finding the Lesson in the Conflict: Personal Growth and Self-Discovery

Conflicts are an inevitable part of life, and they can be incredibly challenging to navigate. However, conflicts also offer us a unique opportunity for personal growth and self-discovery. In this chapter, we will explore how to find the lesson in the conflict and use it as a catalyst for personal growth and self-discovery.

The first step in finding the lesson in the conflict is to approach the situation with a willingness to learn and grow. This means being open-minded, curious, and non-judgmental. It's essential to recognize that conflicts are not about winning or losing but about understanding and learning.

Once we approach the conflict with a willingness to learn, we can begin to identify the lesson. This involves reflecting on our actions, behaviors, and reactions during the conflict. We need to ask ourselves questions like:

- What triggered my reaction?
- How did I respond to the situation?
- What were my motivations and intentions?
- What did I learn about myself and the other person?

By reflecting on these questions, we can gain valuable insights into our thoughts, feelings, and behaviors. We may discover patterns, habits, or areas where we need to improve. This self-awareness is essential for personal growth and self-discovery.

Another crucial step in finding the lesson in the conflict is to practice self-reflection and introspection. This involves taking time to examine our thoughts, feelings, and actions. We need to be honest with ourselves and acknowledge our mistakes and weaknesses. This self-reflection will help us to identify areas where we need to improve and grow.

In addition to self-reflection, it's essential to seek feedback from others. This can be a challenging step, but it's crucial for personal growth and self-discovery. We need to be open to constructive criticism and use it as an opportunity to learn and grow.

Finally, finding the lesson in the conflict requires us to be patient and compassionate with ourselves. We need to recognize that personal growth and self-discovery are lifelong processes. It's essential to be gentle with ourselves and acknowledge that we are doing the best we can.

Conflicts are not just challenges to be overcome but also opportunities for personal growth and self-discovery. By approaching conflicts with a willingness to learn, reflecting on our actions and behaviors, practicing self-reflection and introspection, seeking feedback from others, and being patient and compassionate with ourselves, we can find the lesson in the conflict and use it as a catalyst for personal growth and self-discovery.

Remember, conflicts are not about winning or losing but about understanding and learning. By embracing this mindset, we can transform conflicts into opportunities for personal growth and self-discovery.

CHAPTER FIVE: BUILDING A CULTURE OF BLISS

Creating a Safe and Supportive Relationship Environment

Relationships are a vital part of our lives, and creating a safe and supportive relationship environment is essential for building trust, intimacy, and connection with our partners. In this chapter, we will explore the importance of creating a safe and supportive relationship environment and provide practical tips on how to achieve it.

Why a Safe and Supportive Relationship Environment is Important

A safe and supportive relationship environment is crucial for building trust, intimacy, and connection with our partner. When we feel safe and supported, we are more likely to be our authentic selves, share our thoughts and feelings, and be vulnerable with our partners. This, in turn, creates a deeper sense of connection and intimacy in the relationship.

Characteristics of a Safe and Supportive Relationship Environment

A safe and supportive relationship environment has several key characteristics, including:

- Emotional safety: feeling comfortable sharing thoughts and feelings without fear of judgment or rejection

- Physical safety: feeling comfortable and secure in the physical presence of our partner

- Trust: believing that our partner has our best interests at heart and will be honest and transparent with us

- Respect: feeling valued and respected by our partner

- Empathy: feeling understood and supported by our partner

- Open communication: feeling comfortable sharing thoughts and feelings and listening to our partner's perspective

Practical Tips for Creating a Safe and Supportive Relationship Environment

Creating a safe and supportive relationship environment requires effort and commitment from both partners. Here are some practical tips to help you achieve it:

- Practice active listening: listen carefully to your partner's thoughts and feelings and show that you understand and care

- Be present: be fully present in the moment and put away distractions like phones and TVs

- Show empathy: try to understand your partner's perspective and show that you care

- Be respectful: treat your partner with respect and kindness, even in difficult moments

- Communicate openly: share your thoughts and feelings openly and honestly with your partner

- Be trustworthy: be honest and transparent with your partner and follow through on your commitments

Creating a safe and supportive relationship environment is essential for building trust, intimacy, and connection with our partner. By understanding the characteristics of a safe and supportive relationship environment and practicing the practical tips outlined in this chapter, you can create a relationship that is built on trust, respect, and empathy.

Remember, relationships take work and commitment, but the rewards are well worth it. By creating a safe and supportive relationship environment, you can build a strong and healthy relationship that will bring joy and fulfillment to your life.

The Power of Appreciation and Gratitude in Relationships

Appreciation and gratitude are two of the most powerful tools we have for building strong, healthy relationships. When we focus on appreciating and being grateful for our partner, we create a positive and supportive environment that fosters growth, trust, and intimacy.
We will explore the power of appreciation and gratitude in relationships and provide practical tips on how to cultivate these qualities in your relationships.

Why Appreciation and Gratitude are Important in Relationships

Appreciation and gratitude are essential in relationships because they help us to:

- Focus on the positive aspects of our partner and the relationship
- Build trust and intimacy
- Foster a sense of connection and closeness
- Encourage open and honest communication
- Develop a more optimistic and supportive attitude

Practical Tips for Cultivating Appreciation and Gratitude in Relationships

Here are some practical tips for cultivating appreciation and gratitude in your relationships:

- Practice mindfulness: take time to focus on the present moment and appreciate the small things in your relationship

- Show gratitude: express your gratitude for your partner and the relationship through words, actions, and gestures

- Celebrate milestones: celebrate the big and small milestones in your relationship to show your appreciation and gratitude

- Write love notes: write notes, emails, or texts to your partner to express your appreciation and gratitude

- Give gifts: give gifts that represent your appreciation and gratitude for your partner and the relationship

Appreciation and gratitude are powerful tools for building strong, healthy relationships. By focusing on the positive aspects of our partner and the relationship, we create a supportive environment that fosters growth, trust, and intimacy. Remember, relationships take work and commitment, but the rewards are well worth it.

By cultivating appreciation and gratitude in your relationships, you can build a strong and healthy relationship that will bring joy and fulfillment to your life.

Additionally, you can also include some quotes, anecdotes, or real-life examples to make the content more engaging and relatable.

Sustaining Connection and Intimacy in the Long Term

As we navigate the ups and downs of life, it's easy to let our relationships take a backseat. However, sustaining connection and intimacy in the long term is crucial for building a strong and healthy partnership. In this chapter, we'll explore the importance of connection and intimacy and provide practical tips on how to sustain them in the long term.

Why Connection and Intimacy Matter

Connection and intimacy are the foundation of any successful relationship. They help us build trust, understanding, and a deep sense of bonding with our partner. When we feel connected and intimate, we feel seen, heard, and valued.

However, as time passes, it's easy to let the demands of daily life get in the way of our relationship. We get busy with work,

family, and other obligations, and before we know it, we're feeling disconnected and distant from our partner.
The Consequences of Disconnection

Disconnection can have serious consequences on our relationship. When we feel disconnected, we may start to feel:

- Resentful and angry
- Unheard and unseen
- Unappreciated and unvalued
- Distant and detached

This can lead to a breakdown in communication, trust, and intimacy. It's essential to prioritize connection and intimacy in our relationship to avoid these consequences.

Practical Tips for Sustaining Connection and Intimacy

Here are some practical tips for sustaining connection and intimacy in the long term:

- Schedule regular date nights
- Practice active listening and empathy
- Show appreciation and gratitude
- Engage in activities that bring you joy and closeness
- Practice intimacy and physical touch
- Communicate openly and honestly
- Make time for regular check-ins and connection

Sustaining connection and intimacy in the long term requires effort and commitment from both partners. By prioritizing connection and intimacy, we can build a strong and healthy partnership that brings joy and fulfillment to our lives. Remember, relationships take work, but the rewards are well worth it. By following these practical tips, you can sustain connection and intimacy in the long term and build a relationship that lasts a lifetime.

CHAPTER SIX: PUTTING IT ALL TOGETHER

Conflict to Bliss: The Journey from Separation to Union

Conflict is a natural part of any relationship. It's how we navigate those conflicts that can make or break our connection with our partner. In this chapter, we'll explore the journey from separation to union, and how conflicts can be a catalyst for growth and deeper connection.

The Separation

Separation is a natural part of the relationship cycle. It's the point where we feel disconnected, unheard, and unseen by our partners. This can be a challenging and painful experience, but it's also an opportunity for growth and reflection.

During this phase, we may feel:
- Disconnected and distant from our partner
- Unheard and unseen
- Unappreciated and unvalued
- Angry and resentful

The Conflict

Conflict is the spark that ignites the journey from separation to union. It's the catalyst that forces us to confront our issues, communicate our needs, and work toward a resolution.
During this phase, we may feel:
- Angry and defensive
- Hurt and resentful
- Frustrated and helpless
- Scared and uncertain

The Journey to Union

The journey to union is the process of working through our conflicts and coming out stronger on the other side. It's the process of:

- Communicating our needs and desires
- Listening actively and empathetically
- Working through our issues and finding a resolution
- Rebuilding trust and intimacy

During this phase, we may feel:

- Heard and seen
- Valued and appreciated
- Connected and intimate
- Loved and cherished

The Bliss

The bliss is the culmination of the journey from separation to union. It's the feeling of deep connection, love, and intimacy that comes from working through our conflicts and emerging stronger on the other side.

During this phase, we may feel:
- Deeply connected and intimate
- Loved and cherished
- Valued and appreciated
- Happy and fulfilled

Conflict is not the end of a relationship, but rather a catalyst for growth and deeper connection. By navigating the journey from separation to union, we can emerge stronger, more in love, and more connected than ever before. Remember, relationships take work, but the rewards are well worth it. By working through our conflicts and communicating our needs, we can create a relationship that is built on trust, intimacy, and love.

Maintaining Momentum and Embracing the Journey

As we journey through life, it's easy to get caught up in the destination and forget about the importance of the journey. We set goals and work towards them, but often forget to enjoy the process and celebrate our progress along the way. Lets explore the importance of maintaining momentum and embracing the journey, and provide practical tips on how to do so.

The Importance of Momentum

Momentum is the driving force behind our progress and success. It's the energy and motivation that keeps us moving forward, even when the going gets tough. Without momentum, we can feel stuck and stagnant, like we're not making progress towards our goals.

Momentum is important because it:

- Helps us stay focused and motivated
- Builds confidence and self-belief
- Creates a sense of accomplishment and pride
- Encourages us to take risks and try new things
- Helps us develop a growth mindset

The Journey, Not the Destination

While the destination is important, it's the journey that makes us stronger, wiser, and more resilient. The journey is where we learn and grow, where we face challenges and overcome them. It's where we develop our skills and knowledge, and where we build meaningful relationships with others.

The journey is important because it:

- Helps us develop a sense of purpose and meaning
- Allows us to learn and grow from our experiences
- Builds our character and resilience

- Creates lasting memories and experiences
- Helps us develop a greater appreciation for life

Practical Tips for Maintaining Momentum and Embracing the Journey

Here are some practical tips for maintaining momentum and embracing the journey:

- Set clear and achievable goals
- Break down big goals into smaller, manageable tasks
- Create a schedule and stick to it
- Track your progress and celebrate your successes
- Embrace challenges and view them as opportunities for growth
- Practice self-care and prioritize your well-being
- Surround yourself with positive and supportive people
- Stay focused and motivated by finding your why

Maintaining momentum and embracing the journey is crucial for our success and happiness. By focusing on the process and enjoying the journey, we can build momentum and make progress towards our goals. Remember, the journey is just as important as the destination, and it's where we learn and grow the most. By following these practical tips, you can maintain momentum embrace the journey, and live a life that is fulfilling and meaningful.

EPILOGUE

The Surprising Path to Deeper Love: A Final Word

As we conclude this journey through the surprising path to deeper love, we are reminded that love is a complex and multifaceted emotion that can bring both joy and pain. Yet, it is precisely this vulnerability that makes love so worth pursuing.

In the beginning, we may have thought that love was a destination, a feeling that we could attain and hold onto forever. But as we delved deeper into the journey, we discovered that love is not a static state, but a dynamic process that requires effort, commitment, and growth.

We learned that love is not just a feeling, but a choice that we must make every day. It is a choice to prioritize our partner's needs, to listen actively, to communicate openly, and to embrace each other's imperfections. It is a choice to cultivate intimacy, to build trust, and to create a safe and supportive environment for each other to grow.

We also discovered that love is not just about romance, but about building a deep and meaningful connection with another person. It is about creating a partnership that is based on mutual respect, trust, and understanding. It is about supporting each other's dreams, aspirations, and goals, and about being there for each other through life's ups and downs.

As we reflect on our journey, we may realize that the path to deeper love was not always easy. We may have faced challenges, obstacles, and setbacks along the way. We may have had to confront our fears, insecurities, and limitations. But it is precisely in these moments that we discover our strength, resilience, and capacity for growth.

And so, as we conclude this journey, we are left with a deeper understanding of what it means to love and be loved. We are left with a greater appreciation for the beauty, complexity, and messiness of human relationships. And we are left with a renewed commitment to cultivating deeper love in our own lives, not just with our romantic partners, but with ourselves, our friends, our family, and our community.

In the end, the surprising path to deeper love is not just about finding the perfect partner or achieving a certain level of intimacy. It is about becoming the best version of ourselves, and about creating a life that is filled with purpose, meaning, and connection. It is about embracing the journey, with all its twists and turns, and about trusting that the path will lead us to where we need to be.

And so, dear reader, we bid you farewell, but not goodbye. We know that the journey to deeper love is a lifelong journey and that the path will continue to unfold before us, full of surprises, challenges, and growth opportunities. May you continue to walk this path with courage, curiosity, and an open heart. May you continue to cultivate deeper love in your own life, and may you inspire others to do the same. In the end, it is not just about our journey, but about creating a world that is more loving, compassionate, and connected.